RAISING STRONG GIRLS IN A DIGITAL AGE

Nurturing Resilience in a Time of Change

Deidre Peak

Introduction: Raising Girls in the Digital Age - A Compass for Cultivating Courage and Confidence

The world our daughters are inheriting is a whirlwind of dizzying change. Technology spins on its axis, devouring and birthing new trends faster than we can blink. Social landscapes morph with the swipe of a thumb, leaving yesterday's norms as fossilized relics in the digital dust. It's enough to make any parent, however seasoned, feel like they're steering a sailboat into a hurricane with a map drawn on parchment.

Raising girls in this tech-drenched landscape presents a unique set of challenges and opportunities. From navigating the complex terrain of social media to protecting their developing minds from the pitfalls of hyper-connectivity, we become both expeditionary guides and fierce protectors. But beneath the tech's seductive glow lies a fundamental truth: the human heart, with its yearning for connection, courage, and confidence, remains unchanged. This is where our compass, as parents and caregivers, becomes crucial.

Our journey begins with acknowledging the physical and emotional hurdles girls face in this digital age. Body image distortion, fueled by a relentless barrage of airbrushed ideals, can leave them feeling like imperfect pixels in a flawless filter. Cyberbullying, a venomous whisperer in the digital shadows, can inflict deep wounds on their self-esteem. And the constant pressure to perform, to curate picture-perfect lives online, can lead to anxiety and exhaustion, robbing them of the joy of simply being.

But amidst these challenges lie seeds of incredible resilience. As parents, we must be the gardeners, nurturing these seeds with the sunlight of our understanding and the gentle rain of our empathy. We need to build fortresses of self-esteem, brick by brick, by celebrating their individual strengths and talents, their quirks and curiosities. We must teach them to be the curators of their own stories, not the algorithms behind the filters. And most importantly, we must remind them that their worth is not measured in likes or followers, but in the depth of their compassion, the fire of their spirit, and the kindness in their eyes.

The social landscape our daughters traverse is as intricate as a spiderweb, spun with threads of friendship, rivalry, and unspoken expectations. They navigate cliques and gossip circles, the sting of exclusion as sharp as a broken friendship bracelet. Here, our role becomes that of a patient cartographer, helping them decipher the social map, teaching them the art of setting boundaries, and fostering genuine connections built on shared values and mutual respect. We must equip them with the tools to navigate conflict with grace and assertiveness, reminding them that their voice matters, that their opinions deserve to be heard, and that they have the right to walk away from situations that don't nourish their spirit.

But navigating the complexities of the digital age isn't solely about protecting our daughters from its shadows. It's also about harnessing its immense potential as a tool for empowerment and connection. It can be a platform for their creativity, a stage for their voices to be heard, a window to diverse cultures and perspectives. We can empower them to become digital citizens, responsible and informed navigators of this virtual world. We can teach them to code, to create, to share their passions with the world, and to use technology as a force for good.

Ultimately, raising girls in the digital age is about cultivating inner strength and confidence. It's about reminding them that they are the architects of their own happiness, the authors of their own stories. It's about instilling in them a sense of personal integrity, a belief in their own agency, and the courage to stand tall even when the world feels like it's spinning out of control.

This journey won't be easy. There will be stumbles and setbacks, tears and tantrums. But with a steady hand, an open heart, and a shared compass, we can guide our daughters through the digital jungle, not by shielding them from every thorn, but by equipping them with the tools to navigate it with resilience, grace, and an unwavering belief in their own strength and purpose.

Remember, our daughters are not pixels on a screen. They are daughters of the universe, woven from stardust and possibility. It's our privilege, our responsibility, and our greatest adventure to help them write their own extraordinary stories in the ever-evolving tapestry of the digital age.

This chapter is just the beginning of our journey. In the chapters that follow, we will delve deeper into specific challenges and opportunities, offering practical strategies, real-life anecdotes, and expert insights to guide you on this important path. We will explore topics like building healthy self-esteem, fostering digital literacy, navigating social media, and nurturing girls' inner strength and confidence. Together, we can equip our daughters with the tools they need to not only survive, but thrive, in the dynamic and ever-changing world they inherit.

So, let's take a deep breath, adjust our compasses, and embark on this adventure with open hearts and steady hands. As we navigate the digital wilderness, remember, we are not alone. We have a community of parents, educators, and mentors supporting us, sharing our joys and anxieties, and walking alongside us on this journey. Let us lean on each other, draw strength from each other's experiences, and celebrate each other's victories. Together, we can create a world where our daughters not only survive, but soar, their wings painted with the colours of courage, kindness, and unwavering self-belief.

This is not just a journey for our daughters, but for ourselves as well. As we guide them through the digital labyrinth, we confront our own anxieties, revisit our relationships with technology, and rediscover the magic of human connection in a world obsessed with pixels. It's an opportunity to grow alongside them, to learn from their digital fluency, and to embrace the ever-changing landscape with open eyes and an open mind.

So, let the adventure begin. Let the laughter resonate through the online world, let the tears cleanse the sting of exclusion, let the acts of kindness ripple across the virtual waves. Let us raise a generation of girls who are unafraid to be themselves, who embrace their vulnerabilities as strengths, and who use technology as a tool to connect, create, and make the world a more beautiful place. Let us become the generation that bridges the digital divide, not with fear and skepticism, but with understanding, love, and a shared promise to illuminate the path for our daughters, so they may shine brighter than any filter could ever dream.

This is the legacy we write, not in pixels and hashtags, but in the courage we instill, the love we share, and the unwavering belief in the extraordinary potential of every girl who stands poised on the precipice of the digital age. Let us go forth, then, with open hearts and steady compasses, ready to guide them not just through the wilderness, but to the stars themselves.

This, my friends, is the true adventure of raising girls in the digital age. It's a story waiting to be written, a masterpiece in the making, a symphony of laughter and tears, challenges and triumphs, played out on the ever-evolving stage of our interconnected world. So, let's pick up our pens, tune our instruments, and prepare to be amazed by the beauty and brilliance of our daughters, the architects of their own destinies, the digital queens of a world waiting to be redefined.

This chapter, this book, is not just a guide, it's a declaration. A declaration of our unwavering faith in the future, in the power of connection, and in the boundless potential of the human spirit, embodied in every girl who steps into the digital dawn. As we raise them, we raise ourselves, we raise the world, one pixel of courage, one byte of kindness, one line of code at a time. For in their success, lies our own, in their journey, lies the path to a brighter tomorrow. So, let's walk it together, parents, daughters, hand in hand, hearts ablaze, ready to write the most extraordinary chapter of all.

Chapter 1: Demystifying Puberty: Openly Discussing Physical Changes, Body Image, and Self-Acceptance

Puberty. The mere mention of the word can evoke a chorus of groans, eye rolls, and nervous giggles from both parents and children. It's a time of awkward bumps, hormonal surges, and an emotional rollercoaster that rivals any theme park ride. Yet, beneath the surface of awkward silences and slammed bedroom doors lies a profound transformation, a metamorphosis from child to young adult, a journey etched with physical changes, emotional complexities, and the delicate dance of self-acceptance.

For our daughters, navigating this journey can be daunting. Their bodies, once familiar playgrounds, morph into uncharted territories. Breasts sprout, hips widen, and curves bloom in unexpected places. Hair sprouts in new locations, skin erupts in protest, and voices crack with the uncertainty of their newfound depth. It's a symphony of change, beautiful and bewildering in equal measure.

As parents, our role becomes both crucial and delicate. We are the translators of this biological code, the interpreters of the confusing whispers between hormones and emotions. We are the architects of safe spaces where open dialogue can flourish, where questions, however embarrassing, can be met with patient understanding and reassuring honesty.

But how do we broach these sensitive topics without eliciting cringes or triggering meltdowns? Here are some key approaches:

Start Early: Don't wait for the first awkward question or the blooming of breasts to initiate the conversation. Lay the groundwork early, with age-appropriate explanations about bodies, growth, and the natural rhythms of life. Use relatable analogies, picture books, and even dolls to illustrate the changes that lie ahead. Remember, knowledge is power, and early, open communication can dispel fear and foster understanding.

Normalize the Changes: Puberty is not a disease to be cured or a secret to be hidden. It's a normal, healthy process that every human being experiences. Normalize the physical changes by talking about them matter-of-factly, using accurate and appropriate terminology. Celebrate milestones, like the first period or the growth spurt, as signs of progress and development. This helps our daughters view their bodies not as battlegrounds, but as vessels of change and potential.

Embrace Positive Body Image: The media bombards us with unrealistic ideals of beauty, airbrushed figures that bear little resemblance to the beautiful diversity of real bodies. Counteract this influence by celebrating the unique beauty of your daughter's individual form. Point out her strengths, her quirky features, the way her eyes sparkle when she laughs. Encourage her to find healthy role models who represent a spectrum of body types and ethnicities. Help her cultivate a love for her body, not in spite of its imperfections, but for all its magnificent quirks and capabilities.

Create a Safe Space for Questions: Remember, there are no "silly" questions when it comes to puberty. Be available, approachable, and most importantly, a good listener. Let your daughter know that she can come to you with any question, no matter how embarrassing or uncomfortable it may seem. Create a space where she feels safe to express her anxieties, fears, and hopes about the changes she's experiencing. This open communication builds trust and strengthens your bond, ensuring that she knows she's not alone on this journey.

Focus on Health and Well-being: Puberty is not just about physical changes; it's also a time of emotional and social development.

Encourage healthy habits, like nutritious meals, regular exercise, and adequate sleep. These not only support physical development but also contribute to emotional stability and resilience. Talk about healthy relationships, boundaries, and consent, empowering your daughter to navigate the social landscape with confidence and respect.

Celebrate the Journey: Puberty may be a bumpy road, but it's also a time of tremendous growth and potential. Celebrate the milestones, the newfound independence, the blossoming talents and interests. Remind your daughter that she is worthy, capable, and deserving of love and respect, no matter what changes her body goes through.

Remember, you are not alone on this journey. There are a wealth of resources available, from books and websites to support groups and counseling services. Don't hesitate to seek professional help if you feel overwhelmed or unsure how to handle specific challenges.

By demystifying puberty, fostering open communication, and celebrating the beauty and complexity of this transformative time, we can empower our daughters to navigate this journey with confidence, self-acceptance, and a deep appreciation for the incredible beings they are becoming. So, let's approach puberty not with fear or trepidation, but with curiosity, compassion, and a shared sense of wonder at the magic of human transformation.

Together, we can help our daughters blossom into strong, confident women who embrace their unique bodies and navigate the world with open hearts and empowered voices. They will rise above the noise of unrealistic expectations, celebrate their strengths and diversity, and leave their own indelible mark on the world. Remember, this journey, with all its bumps and beautiful transformations, is not just about our daughters; it's about our own growth as parents, our ability to adapt and learn, and ultimately, our shared faith in the resilience and potential of the human spirit. So, let us embark on this adventure together, hand in hand, with open hearts and ready smiles, prepared to guide, support, and celebrate our daughters as they write their own extraordinary chapters in the story of their lives.

This chapter is not just about puberty, it's about a fundamental shift in perspective. It's about moving from fear and trepidation to acceptance and celebration. It's about recognizing that puberty is not a problem to be solved, but a journey to be embraced. It's about understanding that our daughters are not fragile dolls to be protected, but powerful young women to be empowered.

And so, let us empower them. Let us equip them with the tools of self-acceptance, body positivity, and emotional intelligence. Let us open doors of opportunity, not walls of fear. Let us be their cheerleaders, their confidantes, their guides on this journey of self-discovery. For in their empowerment lies our own, in their success lies the promise of a brighter future, and in their courage and joy, we find the true meaning of raising girls in today's ever-changing world.

This is not just a chapter, it's a declaration. A declaration of our unwavering support for our daughters, our commitment to understanding their challenges, and our belief in their limitless potential. It's a promise to walk with them through the rain and sunshine, to celebrate their victories and pick them up after stumbles, and to be their constant allies in the face of doubt and negativity.

Let us raise a generation of girls who are unafraid to be themselves, who embrace their vulnerabilities as strengths, and who use their voices to challenge the status quo and redefine the very meaning of beauty and success. Let us raise girls who understand that their bodies are not battlegrounds, but instruments of creation, connection, and self-expression.

This is the legacy we leave behind, not in pixelated images or filtered selfies, but in the courage we instill, the love we share, and the unwavering belief in the extraordinary spirit of every girl who stands poised on the precipice of womanhood. As we raise them, we raise ourselves, we raise the world, one step at a time, one conversation at a time, one milestone celebrated with a smile and a hug.

For in their journey lies our own, in their empowerment lies our hope, and in their unwavering spirit, we find the strength to rewrite the narrative, redefine the meaning of beauty, and create a world where every girl, every woman, shines brighter than any filter could ever dream.

So let the adventure begin. Let the conversations flow, let the tears cleanse, let the laughter echo through the halls. Let us be the architects of a world where puberty is not a whispered secret, but a celebrated journey, and where every girl is empowered to embrace the magic of her own becoming. This is our story, our daughters' story, a story waiting to be written, a chapter waiting to be filled with courage, acceptance, and the boundless potential of the human spirit.

Chapter 2: Unfurling Wings: Understanding Emotional Shifts, Mood Swings, And Developing Healthy Coping Mechanisms

As our daughters navigate the tumultuous terrain of puberty, their emotional landscape often resembles a weather map caught in a perpetual storm. Sunny skies of contentment can abruptly darken with clouds of anger, frustration, and tears. One moment they're giggling butterflies, the next, brooding thunderclouds ready to unleash a downpour of negativity. These dramatic shifts, while perplexing and sometimes exhausting for parents, are a normal part of this transformative phase.

Driven by the hormonal rollercoaster within, their emotions dance a wild jig, often leaving them feeling like helpless passengers on a runaway train. The once stable ground of childhood melts away, replaced by a shifting landscape of anxieties, insecurities, and newfound desires. It's a time of questioning everything – their identity, their relationships, their place in the world.

As parents, our role becomes akin to that of seasoned meteorologists, learning to read the subtle signs, interpret the emotional barometric pressure, and equip our daughters with the tools to navigate these emotional storms with resilience and grace.

Understanding the Why: The first step is understanding the "why" behind these volatile emotions. The surge of hormones, particularly estrogen and progesterone, plays a significant role in the emotional upheaval. These hormones act like puppet masters, pulling strings on brain circuits responsible for mood regulation and impulse control. Add to this the cocktail of social pressures, academic demands, and the ever-present quest for identity, and you have a recipe for emotional volatility.

Open Communication is Key: Remember, communication is your life raft in this emotional storm. Create a safe space where your daughter can openly express her anxieties, frustrations, and fears, without judgment or criticism. Active listening, with minimal interruptions and genuine empathy, helps her feel heard and understood. Validate her feelings, even if you don't always agree with them. Remind her that it's okay to feel a range of emotions, and that these feelings are temporary, like passing clouds on a summer sky.

Developing Healthy Coping Mechanisms: Instead of trying to

suppress or shut down their emotions, empower your daughter to develop healthy coping mechanisms. Encourage activities that foster emotional release and self-soothing. Yoga, journaling, nature walks, creative expression through art or music – these are all tools that can help her navigate and process her emotions in a constructive way.

Building Resilience: Teach your daughter the art of resilience. Help her understand that challenges and setbacks are inevitable, but not insurmountable. Equip her with the tools to pick herself up after a fall, dust herself off, and learn from the experience. Encourage positive self-talk, remind her of her strengths and past successes, and help her develop a growth mindset that sees challenges as opportunities for learning and growth.

Setting Boundaries: Setting healthy boundaries, both with herself and others, is crucial for emotional well-being. Teach your daughter to identify situations that trigger her stress or anxiety, and empower her to politely excuse herself or say "no" when needed. Help her establish boundaries in her relationships, teaching her to respect herself and others.

Seeking Support: Sometimes, the emotional storms can feel overwhelming, even for the most equipped of navigators. Encourage your daughter to seek help when needed. Talk to a trusted family member, friend, therapist, or counselor. There is no shame in seeking professional help, and it can be an invaluable resource for navigating the complexities of adolescence.

Remember, our daughters are not simply passengers on this emotional rollercoaster; they are the pilots in training. We equip them with the tools, the emotional radar, and the unwavering belief in their own strength to navigate these storms with confidence and grace. By understanding the "why" behind their emotional shifts, providing a safe space for communication, and equipping them with healthy coping mechanisms, we can help them navigate this critical phase with resilience and emerge on the other side with their wings unfurled, ready to soar.

This journey is not just about weathering the emotional storms; it's about fostering emotional intelligence. It's about teaching our daughters to understand their own emotions, empathize with others, and communicate effectively. It's about equipping them with the tools to manage stress, build healthy relationships, and make responsible choices.

In doing so, we don't just prepare them for the teenage years; we prepare them for life. We create a generation of young women who are emotionally aware, self-confident, and equipped to handle whatever challenges life throws their way. They become not just survivors of the emotional rollercoaster, but architects of their own emotional landscapes, capable of painting their skies with rainbows of resilience and hope.

So let us be their weather forecasters, not with dire warnings and ominous clouds, but with gentle reminders of sunshine and the promise of calmer skies. Let us be their emotional anchors, not by tying them down with expectations, but by offering a steady presence and unwavering support. And let us be their co-pilots on this emotional journey, celebrating celebrating their triumphs over emotional headwinds, offering comfort during turbulence, and cheering them on as they gain altitude, unfurling their wings ever wider. For in their emotional resilience lies our own, in their self-understanding our hope, and in their ability to weather life's storms with grace, we find the strength to rewrite the narrative of adolescence, from chaotic turbulence to a soaring symphony of self-discovery and emotional mastery.

This chapter is not just a map for navigating emotional storms; it's a manifesto for fostering emotional intelligence in our daughters. It's a declaration of our unwavering faith in their emotional capacity, their resilience, and their ability to emerge from this transformative phase not just unscathed, but empowered and brimming with the wisdom gleaned from weathered skies and conquered storms.

Let us raise a generation of girls who understand the power of their emotions, who use them as fuel for creativity and compassion, and who navigate the world with hearts that are both fierce and tender, vulnerable and strong. Let us raise girls who are not afraid to feel, to express, to weather the storms and embrace the calm, for it is in this emotional dance that they discover their true selves, their authentic voices, and the incredible strength that lies within.

This is more than just parenting; it's a revolution of empathy, a rewriting of the narrative around girls' emotions, from fragility to fortitude, from chaos to clarity. In their journey, we find our own, a journey of rediscovering our own emotional landscapes, confronting our anxieties, and learning to navigate life's storms with newfound grace. Together, daughters and parents, hand in hand, we embark on this emotional expedition, not as adversaries, but as adventurers, united by the shared language of the heart, ready to weather any storm and dance upon the rainbow's edge.

So let the tears fall, let the laughter echo, let the anger find its voice, and let the vulnerability bloom. For in this unfurling of emotions lies the extraordinary beauty of being human, the raw power of authenticity, and the promise of a world where girls not only survive, but soar, their emotional wings painting the sky with the vibrant hues of self-discovery and a love for life, in all its glorious, stormy brilliance.

Chapter 3: Friendship Fundamentals: Cultivating Healthy Friendships, Navigating Peer Pressure, And Building Support Networks

As our daughters transition from the sheltered shores of

childhood to the vast and sometimes choppy seas of adolescence, one of the most important anchors they'll grasp onto is friendship. These early bonds with peers nurture their self-esteem, shape their identities, and provide a vital support network as they navigate the complexities of their changing world. Yet, the terrain of friendship in adolescence can be as treacherous as it is rewarding, a landscape strewn with shifting alliances, unspoken rules, and the ever-present pressure to conform.

Therefore, our role as parents becomes akin to seasoned boatwrights, constructing not just a sturdy vessel for these journeys, but also equipping our daughters with the navigational tools to navigate the currents of friendship, avoid the reefs of peer pressure, and chart a course towards healthy, supportive relationships.

Understanding the Importance of Friendship:

For our daughters, friendships are more than just casual playdates or weekend sleepovers. They are crucibles where they experiment with social identities, learn about communication and empathy, and develop vital life skills, like conflict resolution and compromise. Friends become mirrors reflecting back their strengths and weaknesses, confidantes whispering comfort in times of vulnerability, and cheerleaders urging them to reach their full potential. Strong, healthy friendships not only bolster self-esteem, but also serve as protective barriers against negative influences and peer pressure.

Cultivating Healthy Bonds:

So, how do we guide our daughters towards cultivating these healthy, supportive friendships? Here are some key strategies:

- Encourage Diverse Friendships: Remind your daughters that true friends come in all shapes, sizes, and backgrounds.

Diversity not only enriches their lives but also exposes them to different perspectives and fosters acceptance and understanding.

- Teach Communication Skills: Open and honest communication is the bedrock of healthy friendships. Help your daughter build active listening skills, express her needs and feelings assertively, and resolve conflicts constructively.

- Model Healthy Relationships: Our own interactions with friends and family serve as powerful models for our daughters. Demonstrate respect, empathy, and healthy boundaries in your own relationships, offering opportunities for open discussions about conflict resolution and navigating differences.

- Set Ground Rules: Discuss and establish clear expectations regarding online interactions, peer pressure, and acceptable behavior within friendships. These guidelines provide a framework for navigating complex situations and empower your daughter to make responsible choices.

Navigating Peer Pressure:

The relentless tide of peer pressure can be one of the most challenging currents our daughters encounter. The desire to fit in, to be accepted, can tempt them to compromise their values, engage in risky behaviors, or abandon their individuality. Equipping them with the tools to navigate these pressures is crucial for their social and emotional well-being.

- Open Communication is Key: Communication remains the life raft in this choppy water. Create a safe space where your daughter can openly discuss peer pressure situations without judgment. Listen actively, validate her anxieties, and help her explore alternative options.

- Boost Self-Esteem: A strong sense of self-worth serves as a shield against peer pressure. Foster your daughter's unique talents and interests, celebrate her achievements, and remind her of her inherent value, independent of anyone else's approval.

- Role-Playing Scenarios: Practice potential peer pressure situations in a safe, controlled environment. Help your daughter develop assertive communication skills to say "no" confidently and articulate her values without compromising her relationships.
- Build Alternative Support Networks: Encourage your daughter to cultivate a diverse network of friends and positive influences beyond the immediate peer group. This provides a broader circle of support and reinforces her confidence to resist negative pressures.

Building a Support System:

Beyond individual friendships, a strong support system plays a vital role in fostering well-being during adolescence. Encourage your daughter to connect with mentors, coaches, teachers, or extended family members who can offer guidance, encouragement, and alternative perspectives. These connections can be lifelines during challenging times, providing the stability and security that friendships alone might not offer.

Remember, Our Role is to Guide, Not Control:

Throughout this journey, it's crucial to remember that our role is to guide, not control. We can equip our daughters with tools, offer support, and hold a steady hand, but ultimately, the choices they make in navigating the intricate web of friendship are theirs. Trust their instincts, their growing capacity for discernment, and celebrate their victories over social challenges.

Friendship: A Lifelong Voyage:

The friendships our daughters forge in adolescence are not transient alliances, but stepping stones on a lifelong voyage of self-discovery and connection. The lessons learned, the support gained, and the resilience built within these early bonds prepare them to navigate the complex social landscapes of adulthood. As parents, we are not just bystanders on this journey; we are fellow travelers, sharing the joy of laughter, offering comfort in tears, and celebrating the beauty of human connection in its myriad forms.

Remember, the journey of friendship is rarely smooth sailing. There will be storms of misunderstandings, squalls of betrayal, and days when the sun seems hidden by thick clouds of doubt. But it is precisely through these challenges that our daughters develop the strength and resilience needed to navigate the uncharted waters of life.

Our role, then, is not to shield them from these storms, but to equip them with the tools to weather them. We teach them to hoist the sails of communication, anchor themselves in their values, and navigate the currents of conflict with grace and compassion. We remind them that even in the darkest skies, friendship's beacon shines bright, offering guidance, comfort, and the promise of a calmer horizon.

Let us then, be not just navigators, but fellow mariners on this journey. Let us share our own stories of friendship, its joys and tribulations, its bittersweet wisdom and enduring strength. Let us celebrate the laughter echoing across playgrounds, the whispered secrets shared in slumber parties, and the silent understanding that transcends words.

For in the tapestry of friendship, woven with threads of acceptance, loyalty, and shared experiences, our daughters discover not just belonging, but the very essence of humanity. They learn the power of empathy, the beauty of vulnerability, and the strength that comes from being part of something larger than themselves.

And so, let us raise a generation of girls who value friendship not just as a fleeting comfort, but as a compass guiding them through life's storms. Let us raise girls who understand that true friends are not mirrors reflecting back their flaws, but windows opening onto a world of possibilities, a hand outstretched in unwavering support, and a voice whispering courage when the waves threaten to engulf them.

This is not just a chapter on friendship; it's a declaration of faith in the transformative power of human connection. It's a promise to stand by our daughters as they navigate the intricate web of relationships, offering a safe harbor when the seas grow rough and celebrating the shared laughter when the sun breaks through the clouds.

For in their friendships lies our own, in their support networks our strength, and in the enduring bonds they forge, we find the promise of a world not just filled with individuals, but united by the invisible threads of friendship, a world where girls not only survive, but thrive, their wings lifted by the winds of compassion, their sails billowing with the power of connection, and their hearts forever tethered to the anchor of true friendship.

Chapter 4: Social Media Savvy: Setting Boundaries, Promoting Responsible Online Behavior, And Combating Cyberbullying

The digital age has ushered in a new frontier in the landscape of adolescence. Social media, once a novelty, has become an ubiquitous playground, a bustling marketplace of ideas, and a double-edged sword for our daughters. It offers unparalleled opportunities for connection, creativity, and self-expression, yet it also harbors hidden dangers like cyberbullying, privacy concerns, and the relentless pressure to conform to unrealistic ideals. As navigators on this uncharted digital terrain, our role becomes one of equipping our daughters with the tools and awareness to become not just passive consumers, but confident, responsible netizens.

Understanding the Allure and the Risks:

Social media platforms, with their curated feeds and dopamine-inducing algorithms, have a magnetic pull on young minds. They offer a sense of belonging, instant gratification, and a platform for self-discovery. However, it's crucial to acknowledge the inherent risks – cyberbullying, privacy violations, unrealistic beauty standards, and the potential for addiction. Our daughters need to understand that the online world is just one facet of their identity, not the totality of their existence.

Setting Boundaries and Guidelines:

Open communication is paramount in navigating this digital ocean. Discuss expectations and establish clear boundaries regarding online activity. Set time limits, discourage unrestricted access to age-inappropriate content, and discuss the importance of privacy settings and cyber hygiene. Remember, trust is earned, not imposed. Encourage open dialogue about their online experiences, both positive and negative, and create a safe space for them to voice concerns without fear of judgment.

Promoting Digital Citizenship:

Being socially savvy online goes beyond merely following rules. It's about cultivating responsible digital citizenship. Teach your daughters to respect themselves and others online, to think critically about the information they encounter, and to be mindful of their digital footprint. Encourage empathy and responsible communication, reminding them that the anonymity of the screen doesn't absolve them of accountability for their words and actions.

Navigating Cyberbullying:

Cyberbullying, an insidious form of online harassment, can have devastating consequences for young minds. Equip your daughters with the tools to recognize and deal with cyberbullying effectively. Discuss warning signs, teach them to document and report online abuse, and emphasize the importance of seeking help from adults they trust. Remind them that they are not alone, and that cyberbullies do not define their worth or value.

Building Resilience and Fostering Self-Esteem:

The constant barrage of unrealistic beauty standards on social media can wreak havoc on young girls' self-esteem. Help your daughters cultivate a healthy body image by focusing on health, inner beauty, and self-acceptance. Discuss the curated nature of online content, promote positive role models who celebrate diversity, and encourage activities that foster self-love and appreciation for their unique bodies and talents.

Empowering Digital Creators:

Social media can be a powerful tool for self-expression and creativity. Encourage your daughters to use their platforms for positive purposes, whether it's promoting social causes, showcasing their passions, or connecting with like-minded individuals. Guide them towards creating meaningful content that reflects their authentic selves, not chasing likes or conforming to online trends.

Remember, We're Co-Pilots, Not Dictators:

Our role in this digital landscape is not to impose absolute control, but to guide and empower. Equip our daughters with the tools and awareness to navigate this unfamiliar territory safely and responsibly. Remember, trust and open communication are our most potent weapons against the pitfalls of social media.

Beyond Likes and Followers:

Social media, for all its allure and challenges, is just one chapter in the grand narrative of our daughters' lives. The true joy lies not in the number of followers or the curated perfection of their profiles, but in the real-world connections, the authentic experiences, and the meaningful contributions they make to the world around them.

Let us raise a generation of girls who are not just digital consumers, but responsible creators, who use technology as a tool for good, a platform for self-expression, and a bridge to connect with the world around them. Let us foster digital savvy that prioritizes kindness, critical thinking, and self-respect over fleeting trends and superficial interactions.

In this digital age, our daughters hold the potential to rewrite the narrative, to redefine online spaces as arenas for empathy, creativity, and positive change. We, as their guides and companions on this digital journey, can empower them to navigate the currents of social media with confidence, responsibility, and a sense of purpose that extends far beyond the pixels and the screen.

For in their digital citizenship lies our own, in their responsible online behavior our hope, and in their ability to harness technology for good, we find the promise of a world where social media, instead of a battleground, becomes a vibrant tapestry woven with threads of connection, creativity, and a shared pursuit of a better future.

So let the glow not with empty vanity, but with the flickering flames of creativity and compassion. Let the keyboards click not with the hollow echoes of conformity, but with the bold strokes of individual voices and meaningful ideas. Let the digital squares not frame faces contorted in envy, but windows showcasing the beauty of diversity and the boundless potential of the human spirit.

This is not just a chapter on social media; it's a call to action, a manifesto for empowered online citizenship. It's a declaration of faith in our daughters' ability to navigate the digital waves with grace, resilience, and a unwavering commitment to using technology for good. We, as their parents, their teachers, their mentors, stand beside them, not as gatekeepers, but as fellow voyagers, sharing the compass of trust, the map of critical thinking, and the compass star of ethical behavior.

Together, let us embark on this digital odyssey, charting a course towards a future where social media is not a breeding ground for negativity, but a fertile ground for empathy, empowerment, and positive change. Let us raise a generation of girls who are not just savvy consumers of digital trends, but architects of a new online landscape, where connection trumps comparison, where kindness clicks louder than hate, and where the true measure of success is not the number of followers, but the depth of impact they leave on the world around them.

In their digital footprints, we find our own, in their responsible online behavior our hope, and in their ability to rewrite the narrative of social media, we rediscover the power of human connection, the strength of a collective voice, and the promise of a brighter future, both online and off.

Chapter 5: Body And Beauty In The Digital Age: Dismantling Unrealistic Standards, Promoting Self-Love, And Building Body Positivity

For our daughters, navigating the treacherous terrain of

adolescence is already a daunting task. But in the era of the digitized image, where airbrushed perfection reigns and unrealistic beauty standards bombard them from every screen, the journey towards self-acceptance can seem like scaling Mount Everest in flip-flops. Our role, then, becomes akin to Sherpas: guiding them past the dizzying heights of comparison, equipping them with the tools to dismantle societal expectations, and ultimately, helping them plant the flag of self-love on the pinnacle of body positivity.

Unmasking the Mirage of "Perfect" Bodies:

The curated feeds and filtered selfies lining the digital highways whisper insidious messages: flawless skin, impossible curves, and chiseled features become the only acceptable currency of beauty. It's crucial to help our daughters see through this carefully constructed mirage. Discuss the artifice of digital manipulation, expose the unrealistic ideals perpetuated by the media, and remind them that the bodies they see online are often the product of lighting, angles, and a whole lot of editing magic.

Celebrating Diversity, Not Monotony:

Beauty, like a vibrant tapestry, thrives in its diversity. Help your daughters appreciate the kaleidoscope of human forms, the spectrum of skin tones, hair textures, and body shapes that make our world a masterpiece. Expose them to diverse role models – activists, athletes, artists, scientists – who shatter the mold of conventional beauty and redefine what it means to be beautiful. Discuss the harmful effects of comparing themselves to one-dimensional, unattainable ideals, and encourage them to find beauty in their own unique features and the stories their bodies tell.

Planting the Seeds of Self-Love:

Body positivity is not just a hashtag; it's a revolution rooted in self-acceptance and appreciation. Guide your daughters towards cultivating a nurturing relationship with their bodies. Encourage them to focus on health and well-being, engaging in activities that make them feel strong, energized, and capable, rather than chasing impossible aesthetic ideals. Celebrate their strengths, their talents, their resilience, and remind them that their worth is far beyond the confines of their physical form.

Combating the Toxic Influence of "Body Shaming":

The digital battlefield is often rife with negativity, and body shaming can rear its ugly head in comments, memes, and even casual conversations. Equip your daughters with the tools to recognize and dismantle this negativity. Teach them to assert boundaries, report abusive behavior, and surround themselves with people who celebrate their authentic selves. Remind them that they are not defined by the words of others, and that their inner beauty shines brighter than any hurtful comment.

Cultivating Mindfulness and Gratitude:

The constant barrage of images and messages can lead to a hyper-critical internal dialogue. Encourage your daughters to practice mindfulness, shifting their focus from external scrutiny to internal appreciation. Remind them to be grateful for their healthy bodies, the amazing things they can do, and the unique experiences their bodies allow them to have. Gratitude, like a shield, deflects the arrows of self-doubt and fosters a kinder, more accepting relationship with oneself.

Embracing Imperfections:

Perfection is a cruel, elusive butterfly, always just out of reach. Help your daughters embrace their "flaws" and imperfections as part of their story, not detractions from it. Stretch marks, freckles, scars – these are not blemishes, but badges of honor, testaments to a life lived, experiences embraced, and stories etched onto the skin. Teach them to find beauty in the unexpected, celebrating the individuality that makes them who they are.

Remember, We're Mirrors, Not Sculptors:

Our role in this journey is not to mold our daughters into preconceived notions of beauty, but to become mirrors reflecting their inherent worth and celebrating their unique forms. Listen to their anxieties, validate their insecurities, and offer unwavering support as they navigate the turbulent waters of body image. Remember, their journey is their own, and our job is to walk beside them, hand in hand, with lanterns of love and acceptance lighting the way.

Beyond the Pixelated Perfection:

The true beauty of our daughters lies not in the fleeting trends of the digital world, but in the depths of their character, the fire in their souls, and the kindness that radiates from within. It's in their laughter, their compassion, their dreams, and their unwavering spirit. Help them see their bodies as instruments for living, for creating, for connecting, and for making a difference in the world.

Together, let us raise a generation of girls who defy the tyranny of unrealistic beauty standards. Let us raise girls who see their bodies not as battlegrounds, but as vessels of joy, strength, and limitless potential. Let us raise girls who love and celebrate their bodies, in all their glorious, imperfect, magnificent diversity.

For in their self-acceptance lies our own freedom from societal pressures, our own journey towards embracing our individual narratives. In their celebration of diversity, we find the tapestry of humanity beautifully woven, each thread unique and integral to the whole. And in their voices, amplified by body positivity, we hear the call for a world where beauty is not a weapon of exclusion, but a symphony of acceptance, inclusivity, and a love for life in all its messy, breathtaking complexity.

This is not just a chapter on body image; it's a revolution of self-compassion, a manifesto for dismantling the oppressive walls of unrealistic expectations. It's a declaration of faith in our daughters' strength, resilience, and their inherent right to love and appreciate their bodies, not despite their imperfections, but because of them.

We, as mothers, fathers, siblings, mentors, and allies, stand beside them, not as dictators of perfection, but as architects of support, building bridges of understanding, and crafting shelters of acceptance. We offer our stories, our vulnerabilities, and our unwavering belief in their worth, not contingent upon the size of their clothes or the smoothness of their skin.

Together, let us rise as a unified chorus, chanting the vibrant hymns of body positivity, drowning out the discordant whispers of self-doubt. Let us rewrite the narrative, not on pixels and screens, but on the very canvases of our daughters' hearts, with vibrant strokes of self-love, acceptance, and the unwavering belief that they are, in every perfect imperfection, absolutely, undeniably beautiful.

So let the mirrors reflect not unattainable ideals, but the radiant beauty of authentic selves. Let the filters fade, revealing the raw honesty of laughter lines and tear tracks. Let the airbrushed facades crumble, giving way to the kaleidoscope of skin tones, shapes, and sizes that paint the world in magnificent hues.

In this revolution of self-love, we find our own, in their voices our song, and in their acceptance, a world where girls not only survive, but soar, their wings painted with the vibrant colors of self-celebration, leaving a trail of beauty and courage across the digital sky.

Chapter 6: Mental Health Awareness: Recognizing The Whispers Within, Fostering Open Communication, And Building Safe Spaces

As our daughters navigate the tumultuous terrain of adolescence, their emotional landscape can shift like the sands of a desert – vibrant one moment, shadowed the next. While fleeting mood swings are a natural part of this transformative phase, recognizing the deeper whispers of anxiety, depression, or other mental health concerns is crucial for ensuring their well-being. Our role, then, becomes akin to seasoned weather forecasters, learning to read the subtle signs, interpret the emotional barometric pressure, and equip our daughters with the tools to navigate these storms with resilience and support.

Opening the Doors of Communication:

The foundation of navigating any emotional storm is communication. Create a safe space where your daughter feels comfortable expressing her anxieties, frustrations, and fears, without judgment or criticism. Active listening, devoid of interruptions and laced with genuine empathy, can be the lighthouse guiding her through choppy waters. Validate her feelings, even if they differ from your own, reminding her that it's okay to feel a range of emotions, and that these feelings are temporary, like passing clouds on a summer sky.

Recognizing the Shifting Sands:

Mental health concerns often manifest in subtle ways, hiding beneath the surface like seeds waiting to sprout. Be mindful of changes in behavior, sleep patterns, appetite, or energy levels. Persistent sadness, withdrawal from social activities, unexplained anger, or difficulty concentrating can be indicators of deeper struggles. Remember, changes in appearance, either drastic or subtle, can also be a cry for help.

Beyond Labels, Understanding the Landscape:

While recognizing symptoms is crucial, don't get caught in the storm of self-diagnosis. Labels can be limiting, and focusing solely on symptoms can overshadow the unique experiences and emotional complexities of your daughter. Instead, focus on understanding the root causes of her distress, the triggers that fuel her anxieties or the burdens that weigh on her heart. Listen to her story, her fears, her hopes, and use that understanding to build pathways towards support and healing.

Building Bridges of Support:

Remember, you are not alone in this journey. Seek professional help if needed. Therapists, counselors, and school psychologists can provide invaluable guidance and support, not just for your daughter, but for you as well. Navigating mental health concerns can be overwhelming, and having access to professional expertise can equip you with effective tools to address these challenges.

Normalizing the Conversation:

Mental health should not be shrouded in secrecy or shame. Openly discuss mental well-being within your family, creating a space where vulnerability is not weakness, but strength. Share your own experiences, struggles, and victories, highlighting the importance of seeking help and prioritizing emotional well-being. Normalize the conversation around mental health, demonstrating that it is just another facet of our overall health, deserving of attention and care.

Building a Network of Support:

Encourage your daughter to build a strong support network beyond the family unit. Friends, mentors, teachers, or trusted adults can play vital roles in providing a sense of belonging, understanding, and encouragement. Foster connections with individuals who share similar interests or life experiences, creating a web of support that stretches beyond the immediate family circle.

Remember, We're Navigators, Not Rescue Boats:

Our role is not to control or smother our daughters, but to empower them to navigate their own emotional landscape. Equip them with the tools to recognize emotional shifts, communicate effectively, and seek help when needed. Trust their instincts, their inherent resilience, and their capacity to weather these storms.

Beyond the Stormy Skies:

Remember, mental health concerns are not permanent fixtures on the landscape of life. Just as the darkest skies eventually give way to sunshine, emotional struggles can be overcome with the right support and resources. Celebrate victories, both big and small, along the way, reminding your daughter of her strength and her ability to navigate towards calmer waters.

Together, Building a Brighter Future:

By fostering open communication, recognizing the signs of emotional distress, and building a network of support, we can ensure that our daughters are not left alone to weather the storms of mental health. This is not just about supporting individual well-being; it's about creating a generation that understands the importance of mental health, normalizes seeking help, and actively strives to build a world where vulnerability is met with compassion, and emotional struggles are tackled with empathy and understanding.

In their resilience lies our own, in their open communication our hope, and in their ability to access and prioritize their mental well-being, we find the promise of a world where mental health is not a stigma, but a conversation, a journey navigated together, hand in hand, towards a brighter, healthier future, both for our daughters and for ourselves.

So let the tears fall, not as symbols of shame, but as cleansing rain. Let the laughter echo, not as a mask, but as a melody of hope. Let the anxieties whisper their stories, not in the shadows of fear, but in the safe haven of a listening ear. Let the vulnerabilities bloom, not as weeds of weakness, but as flowers of courage, seeking the nourishing rays of acceptance and understanding.

This is not just a chapter on mental health; it's a manifesto for emotional literacy, a blueprint for building bridges of connection instead of walls of isolation. It's a declaration of faith in the inherent strength of our daughters, their capacity for healing, and their right to access the support and resources needed to navigate the ever-shifting landscapes of their minds.

Together, let us raise a generation that speaks the language of emotions, fluent in the vocabulary of vulnerability and adept at navigating the complex currents of mental well-being. Let us be guides, not dictators, offering our hands as anchors in stormy seas, our voices as beacons in the fog, and our hearts as safe harbors where fears can find solace and anxieties can breathe again.

Let us dismantle the stigma brick by brick, building a world where open conversations about mental health flow freely, like rivers nourishing the parched earth. Let us create communities where seeking help is not a whisper of shame, but a resounding chorus of collective support, echoing through schools, homes, and hearts.

In their journeys towards emotional well-being, we find our own, in their resilience our strength, and in their voices, the power to rewrite the narrative of mental health, not as a silent struggle, but as a shared pursuit of wholeness, acceptance, and the unwavering belief that every mind deserves to flourish, bloom, and thrive.

So let the sun break through the clouds, not just on the tapestry of our daughters' lives, but on the collective landscape of a world where mental health is not a battleground, but a garden, tended with love, understanding, and the ever-growing hope that together, we can nurture, heal, and blossom, mind, body, and soul.

Chapter 7: The Big Talk: Navigating The Labyrinth Of Sex, Consent, And Healthy Relationships

The "Big Talk" – that elusive, often dreaded conversation about sex, consent, and healthy relationships. It looms large in the minds of parents, a daunting mountain to climb on the already winding path of adolescence. Yet, avoiding this crucial dialogue is like letting our daughters embark on a perilous journey without a map, leaving them vulnerable to the treacherous terrain of misinformation, peer pressure, and potentially harmful experiences.

So, how do we equip them with the compass of knowledge, the lantern of understanding, and the sturdy boots of self-respect to navigate this complex landscape? Here's our guide to making the "Big Talk" not just big, but meaningful, productive, and, dare we say, even enjoyable.

Setting the Stage for Open Communication:

First, ditch the one-and-done monologue approach. Create a safe space for ongoing, open communication, where your daughter feels comfortable asking questions, expressing curiosity, and voicing her fears without judgment. Build trust and transparency from a young age, talking about emotions, relationships, and boundaries in everyday situations. Remember, this journey starts long before the birds and the bees conversation.

The Language of Understanding:

Terminology matters. Use age-appropriate, accurate language. Don't shy away from technical terms like "vagina," "penis," or "consent," explaining them with clarity and respect. This empowers your daughter to own her body and communicate effectively with partners. Remember, vagueness and euphemisms only muddy the waters, leaving space for confusion and misinformation.

Beyond Anatomy, the Spectrum of Relationships:

The "Big Talk" shouldn't be solely about mechanics. Discuss the emotional and social aspects of relationships. Talk about respect, boundaries, communication, trust, and mutual support. Help your daughter recognize different types of relationships – romantic, platonic, casual, committed – and understand the importance of healthy dynamics within each.

Consent: The Cornerstone of Healthy Relationships:

Consent is not just a word; it's a principle, a foundational pillar of safe and respectful relationships. Make it crystal clear: consent must be enthusiastic, clear, and freely given, every time, for every activity. Discuss scenarios, role-play situations, and emphasize the importance of respecting a "no" at any point, regardless of context or pressure. Remember, silence is not consent, and coercion or manipulation is never acceptable.

Beyond the Biological, Navigating Emotions:

Adolescence is a whirlwind of emotions, and feelings often cloud judgment. Discuss the role of emotions in relationships, both positive and negative. Talk about jealousy, anger, hurt, and disappointment, equipping your daughter with tools to communicate these emotions assertively and navigate conflict constructively.

Breaking the Silence: Addressing Taboos and Misinformation:

Be prepared to tackle uncomfortable topics. Myths and misinformation around sex and relationships abound. Don't shy away from discussing topics like pornography, contraception, sexually transmitted infections, and sexual orientation. Address harmful stereotypes and biases head-on, providing your daughter with accurate information and promoting acceptance and understanding.

Beyond Lectures, Cultivating Critical Thinking:

This is not about dictating rules; it's about empowering your daughter to make informed choices. Encourage critical thinking, skepticism, and open discussion. Challenge her to analyze media messages, question cultural norms, and develop her own values and beliefs around sex and relationships.

Remember, We're Guides, Not Gatekeepers:

Our role is not to control or dictate our daughters' choices, but to guide them towards making responsible decisions for themselves. Trust their inherent wisdom and resilience, while equipping them with the knowledge and tools to navigate challenges. Remember, open communication is a two-way street; listen actively, validate their feelings, and offer non-judgmental support.

Beyond the Talk, Building a Support Network:

The "Big Talk" is not a one-time event; it's an ongoing conversation. Encourage your daughter to seek additional information and support from trusted adults, books, websites, or educational resources. Let her know that she is not alone, and that help and guidance are always available.

Preparing for the Unexpected:

The path of life rarely follows a predictable script. Be prepared to address unexpected situations, like unwanted advances, peer pressure, or unhealthy relationships. Assure your daughter that she can always confide in you, no matter what the issue, and that you will be there to support her and offer guidance.

Remember, We're Navigating Too:

This journey isn't just for our daughters; it's for us as well. Let's be open to learning, revisiting outdated notions, and challenging our own biases. As we guide our daughters, we simultaneously embark on a journey of self-reflection and growth, ensuring that the map we offer is not a dusty relic, but a vibrant, evolving treasure map leading towards a world of healthy relationships built on the bedrock of respect, consent, and mutual understanding.

This is not just a chapter on "The Big Talk"; it's a manifesto for empowering communication, a declaration of faith in our daughters' inherent wisdom, and a call to action for creating a world where sex and relationships are not shrouded in secrecy and shame, but navigated with openness, honesty, and a collective commitment to fostering healthy love and connection.

Together, let us raise a generation with voices that speak clearly about their needs and desires, minds equipped to critically analyze societal norms, and hearts brimming with the empathy and respect needed to build fulfilling, equitable relationships. Let us be not just guides, but co-explorers, venturing into the labyrinth of love and intimacy alongside our daughters, offering not dogmatic pronouncements, but lanterns of understanding, unwavering support, and the unwavering belief that every girl deserves to experience the joy, respect, and empowerment of healthy relationships, both at the tender age of fourteen and far beyond.

For in their choices, we find our own, in their critical thinking our hope, and in their ability to forge healthy connections, we discover the promise of a world not just free from coercion and pain, but filled with the vibrant tapestry of diverse partnerships, woven with threads of empathy, trust, and the shared pursuit of a love that honors the individual yet strengthens the whole.

So let the voices rise, not in whispers of fear, but in choruses of understanding. Let the questions flow, not met with judgment, but with open ears and curious minds. Let the boundaries be set, not as walls of isolation, but as lines of respect and self-care.

In this labyrinth of love and intimacy, let us build bridges of communication, illuminate paths of knowledge, and create a world where our daughters, and ourselves, can navigate the terrain of relationships with confidence, clarity, and the unwavering belief that the journey towards healthy love is not paved with fear, but with the exhilarating potential for joy, fulfillment, and connection that enriches lives and transcends generations.

Chapter 8: The Suicide Talk: Navigating The Shadowlands Of Despair And Illuminating The Path To Hope

There are some conversations we dread – the ones that dance on the precipice of our fears, whispering of darkness we hope never to encounter. The "suicide talk" with our daughter is one such conversation, a conversation both necessary and terrifying. Yet, to shy away from it, to cloak ourselves in silence, is to leave her navigating the labyrinth of despair alone, without the lifeline of our love and the beacon of our understanding.

This chapter is not a roadmap to grief; it's a lantern for courage, a compass for empathy, and a testament to the enduring power of hope in the face of despair. It's a call to action, a plea for open communication, and a guide to creating a safe space where vulnerability isn't punished, but embraced, where whispers of suicide find not judgment, but a chorus of support and a collective commitment to seeking help.

Breaking the Silence:

Suicide, like so many mental health struggles, thrives in the shadows. It whispers in the silence, festers in the unspoken. The first step, then, is to shatter that silence. Talk about suicide openly, frankly, and without fear. Dismantle the stigma, debunk the myths, and create a space where your daughter feels comfortable expressing her emotions, no matter how dark or unsettling they may seem. Remember, mentioning suicide doesn't increase the risk; it opens the door to dialogue, support, and potentially life-saving intervention.

Recognizing the Shadows:

Suicide doesn't appear out of thin air. Be mindful of potential warning signs – changes in behavior, sleep patterns, or appetite, social withdrawal, hopelessness, or expressions of worthlessness. Listen for coded language, phrases like "I wish I wasn't here," "life is pointless," or "no one would miss me." Don't dismiss these as exaggerations or teenage angst; take them seriously and address them with concern and open ears.

Creating a Safe Harbor:

Make it clear that you are a safe space, a harbor where she can weather any storm, even the storms of suicidal ideation. Assure her of your unconditional love and acceptance, regardless of what she reveals. Remember, judgment will only drive her further into the shadows; validate her feelings, listen without interruption, and offer your unwavering support.

Beyond Panic, Taking Action:

The "suicide talk" is not an endpoint; it's a springboard to action. Don't let fear paralyze you. Reach out for professional help. Seek guidance from therapists, counselors, or mental health professionals trained to navigate these delicate situations. Remember, you are not alone in this; there are individuals and resources dedicated to supporting both you and your daughter.

Beyond Diagnosis, Building a Support Network:

Connect your daughter with support networks beyond the therapeutic realm. Encourage her to lean on trusted friends, family members, teachers, or mentors who can offer empathy, understanding, and a sense of belonging. Foster connections with support groups or online communities where she can find solace and connection with others navigating similar struggles.

Remember, We're Life Rafts, Not Rescue Boats:

Our role is not to control or dictate, but to provide a lifeline, a steady presence in the midst of the storm. Empower your daughter to make her own choices, encourage her to seek help, and stand beside her on the journey towards healing. Trust her strength, her resilience, and remember that hope, even in the darkest moments, can be a powerful flame that refuses to be extinguished.

Beyond the Shadows, Illuminating Hope:

This journey through the shadowlands of despair may seem long and arduous, but remember, hope endures. Celebrate victories, both big and small, reminding your daughter of her inherent strength and her capacity to overcome even the most daunting challenges. Share stories of resilience, stories of individuals who emerged from the darkness and found light. Let these stories be testaments to the enduring power of hope, a beacon guiding her towards a brighter future.

Together, Building a Brighter World:

By openly discussing suicide, seeking help, and fostering a culture of support, we can dismantle the stigma surrounding mental health and create a world where vulnerability is met with compassion, and cries for help are answered with a chorus of support. In their journeys towards healing, we find our own, in their resilience our strength, and in their rediscovery of hope, we glimpse the promise of a world where suicide is not a silent killer, but a battle we face together, armed with the tools of communication, empathy, and a collective commitment to saving lives.

So let the tears fall, not as symbols of despair, but as cleansing rain. Let the fears be spoken, not whispered in the dark, but met with the warm embrace of understanding. Let the cries for help ring out, not into the void, but into a chorus of support, a symphony of caring voices raised in unison, declaring that no one shall walk this path alone. Let the darkness be illuminated, not with harsh judgment, but with the gentle glow of compassion and the unwavering belief in the potential for healing.

This is not just a chapter on the "suicide talk"; it's a manifesto for empathy, a declaration of faith in the human spirit's resilience, and a call to action for building communities where suicide prevention is not an afterthought, but a shared responsibility, woven into the very fabric of our social fabric. It's a promise to stand beside our daughters, not just in sunshine, but in the stormiest nights, whispering words of love, lighting lanterns of hope, and reminding them, with every beat of our hearts, that the darkness never conquers the dawn.

Together, let us raise a generation that speaks openly about mental health, a generation that reaches out for help without fear, and a generation that embraces vulnerability as a strength, not a weakness. Let us break the silence, shatter the stigma, and illuminate the path towards a world where suicide is not an ending, but a turning point, a bridge crossed, and a battle won in the name of life, love, and the undying spirit of hope.

In their stories of struggle and survival, we find our own, in their tears our compassion, and in their rediscovered joy, we witness the triumphant dawn of a future where darkness holds no dominion, and every life, like a resilient flame, flickers ever brighter, lighting the way for generations to come.

Chapter 9: Setting Boundaries, Saying No: Cultivating The Courage To Claim Your Space

"No" – a seemingly simple word, yet for our daughters navigating the turbulent waters of adolescence, it can feel like a mountain to climb. In a world that often prizes people-pleasing and societal expectations, asserting boundaries and learning to say no can be a radical act, a reclamation of personal space and a powerful declaration of self-worth. Our role, then, becomes akin to Sherpas on this journey, equipping them with the tools and the courage to confidently claim their space, respect their limits, and build healthy boundaries that protect their emotional and physical well-being.

Beyond the Walls, Building Bridges of Communication:

Healthy boundaries are not walls that isolate; they are bridges that communicate respect, self-worth, and the need for personal space. Encourage open communication around boundaries, discussing their importance and empowering your daughter to articulate her needs assertively. Remember, setting boundaries is not about controlling or manipulating others; it's about clearly communicating your own needs and limitations in a way that fosters mutual respect and understanding.

Know Your "Why": Identifying Your Limits:

Before setting boundaries, help your daughter explore her "why" – the reasons behind her needs and the values she desires to uphold. Is it about protecting her time? Preserving her emotional well-being? Maintaining healthy relationships? Identifying the underlying values strengthens her resolve and empowers her to say no with conviction.

Respecting Yourself, Respecting Others:

Setting boundaries is not about self-centeredness; it's about self-respect. By respecting your own needs and limitations, you demonstrate to your daughter that she too deserves to have her boundaries respected. Encourage her to treat others with the same respect, empowering her to navigate situations where others may try to cross her boundaries.

Beyond Words, The Body Speaks:

Communication goes beyond words; body language plays a crucial role in setting boundaries. Teach your daughter the power of confident eye contact, clear posture, and assertive tone of voice. Help her recognize and address uncomfortable physical contact or situations that violate her sense of personal space.

Navigating the Storm: Saying No in Challenging Situations:

Saying no can be daunting, especially when faced with peer pressure, parental expectations, or societal norms. Role-play challenging situations, empowering your daughter to practice saying no in different contexts. Prepare her for potential pushback and equip her with tools to politely but firmly reiterate her position. Remember, a consistent "no" is stronger than a wavering "maybe."

The Strength of Vulnerability: Setting Boundaries with Loved

Ones:

Setting boundaries with loved ones can be particularly challenging. Encourage your daughter to communicate her needs honestly and openly with family and friends. Remember, setting boundaries doesn't equate to conflict; it can strengthen relationships by establishing clear expectations and fostering mutual respect.

Beyond Labels, Building Healthy Relationships:

Healthy boundaries are not about categorizing people or creating distance; they are about establishing healthy dynamics within relationships. Help your daughter recognize the difference between supportive relationships that respect her boundaries and those that disregard or manipulate her needs. Encourage her to prioritize relationships that foster mutual respect and understanding.

Remember, We're Guides, Not Dictators:

Our role is not to dictate or control our daughters' decisions; it's to equip them with the tools and confidence to make informed choices for themselves. Trust their intuitive wisdom and their evolving understanding of their own needs. Remember, setting boundaries is a lifelong journey, a continuous process of self-discovery and claiming your space in the world.

Beyond Silence, Building a Culture of Respect:

By openly discussing boundaries and supporting our daughters in establishing them, we contribute to building a culture of respect, both within our families and in the wider world. Imagine a world where saying no is not met with judgment, but with understanding, where personal space is not an imposition, but a valued attribute, and where relationships thrive on mutual respect for each other's boundaries.

Together, Building Bridges of Confidence:

In their journeys towards claiming their space, we find our own, in their voices of assertiveness our strength, and in their empowered presence, we witness the construction of a world where girls flourish not despite their boundaries, but because of them, confident, respected, and empowered to live life on their own terms.

So let the voices rise, clear and unwavering, declaring their needs and claiming their space. Let the "no"s be spoken with conviction, not as weapons, but as shields of self-respect. Let the bridges of communication be built, not upon foundations of fear, but upon the bedrock of empathy and mutual understanding.

In this landscape of self-discovery, let us be not dictators, but co-explorers, venturing alongside our daughters, offering unwavering support, celebrating their victories, and reminding them, with every beat of our hearts, that the power to set boundaries, and claim their space in the world, is not just a privilege, but a birthright, an inherent right etched into the very fabric of their being. Let the walls crumble, not just around them, but within ourselves, as we dismantle outdated notions of female passivity and embrace the empowering strength of a girl who knows her worth, respects her limits, and claims her space in the world with the fierce grace of a warrior queen.

Together, let us raise a generation of girls who navigate the labyrinth of life with the unyielding compass of self-respect, their voices strong, their boundaries clear, and their hearts brimming with the unwavering belief that to claim your space is not to shrink, but to expand, to step into the fullness of your potential and illuminate the world with the radiant light of your own unique self.

For in their stories of boundaries set and voices heard, we find our own liberation, in their confidence our inspiration, and in their empowered presence, the promise of a future where girls don't just survive, but thrive, architects of their own destiny, builders of bridges of connection, and champions of a world where respect flows freely, like a river nourishing the parched earth, quenching the thirst for belonging, and washing away the dust of doubt that once obscured the dazzling potential of every girl who dares to say no.

Chapter 10: Raising Responsible Daughters: Cultivating The Garden Of Character

Raising daughters demands more than nurturing their minds and bodies; it calls for tending to the fertile ground of their character, cultivating the seeds of empathy, integrity, and accountability. These values, woven into the tapestry of their being, become the compass guiding them through life's triumphs and challenges, shaping them into individuals of compassion, conscience, and unwavering responsibility for their actions and choices.

Empathy: Sowing the Seeds of Compassion:

Empathy is the cornerstone of responsible action. Help your daughter develop the ability to step outside her own perspective, to imagine the world through another's eyes. Encourage her to actively listen, not just to words, but to emotions unspoken. Foster her curiosity about diverse experiences, cultures, and backgrounds, opening her heart to the tapestry of human emotions woven around her. Let her witness acts of kindness, volunteer in her community, and expose her to stories of resilience and altruism. Allow her to witness your own vulnerabilities and compassion to understand that empathy begins at home.

Integrity: Watering the Roots of Honesty:

Integrity is the unwavering commitment to truth, even when it's difficult. Teach your daughter that honesty is not just a principle, but a muscle that needs constant exercise. Encourage her to speak her truth, even when it means owning up to mistakes or facing consequences. Celebrate her courage to be authentic, and demonstrate the power of integrity in your own words and actions. Remember, hypocrisy wilts the delicate blooms of honesty; strive to align your words with your actions, living as a role model of unwavering integrity.

Accountability: Pruning the Weeds of Blame:

Accountability is the willingness to take ownership of one's actions and choices, both positive and negative. Teach your daughter that mistakes are inevitable, but the path to responsibility lies in owning them, learning from them, and making amends. Foster a safe space where she can admit to slip-ups without fear of judgment, guiding her towards reflection and understanding instead of blame and shame. Remember, blaming others allows the weeds of self-deception to flourish; instead, cultivate the responsibility to take ownership, learn, and grow from every action, creating a fertile ground for accountability to thrive.

Beyond Words, Living the Values:

These values are not mere words to be preached; they are seeds to be planted, nurtured, and allowed to bloom in the everyday garden of your lives. Integrate them into the fabric of your family, making empathy, integrity, and accountability the guiding principles in your interactions with each other and the world around you. Engage in open discussions about ethical dilemmas, celebrate acts of kindness, and hold each other accountable for actions and choices. Remember, your everyday actions speak volumes; let your daughters witness you putting these values into practice, demonstrating how to navigate life with a firm grip on the compass of responsibility.

Weathering the Storms: Nurturing Resilience and Self-Correction:

The journey towards responsible living is not a straight path; it's an uphill climb with twists and turns, storms and sunshine. There will be stumbles, missteps, and moments where empathy dims, integrity wavers, and accountability feels daunting. These are not failures; they are opportunities for growth, chances to strengthen the roots of character and nurture the resilience needed to weather life's storms. Guide your daughter towards self-forgiveness, helping her learn from mistakes and use them as stepping stones for future growth. Remember, every storm nourishes the soil, strengthening the roots and preparing the garden for even more vibrant blooms.

Beyond Limits, Expanding the Circle of Compassion:

Raising responsible daughters isn't just about shaping individuals; it's about planting seeds of change in the wider world. Encourage your daughter to extend her circle of empathy and responsibility beyond her own needs and desires. Foster her engagement with social causes, environmental concerns, and acts of community service. Help her understand that her choices and actions have ripple effects, impacting not just herself but the world around her. Remember, every seed of compassion sown, every act of responsible living, contributes to a world where the garden of character blooms not just within individuals, but in the shared landscape of humanity.

Together, Growing a Forest of Responsibility:

In their journeys towards responsible living, we find our own, in their empathy our connection, and in their unwavering commitment to integrity and accountability, we witness the promise of a brighter future. Together, let us raise daughters who not only navigate life with a compass of responsibility, but cultivate and share these values with others, transforming the landscape of our world into a vibrant forest of empathy, integrity, and a collective commitment to building a world where every individual grows tall, strong, and accountable, reaching towards the sun with the knowledge that their choices, like seeds scattered on fertile ground, have the power to bloom into a more just, compassionate, and responsible future for all.

So let the gardens flourish, not just within them, but outwards, into the community, weaving tendrils of responsibility and compassion that bind us together in a tapestry of shared humanity. Let the roots of empathy burrow deep, nourishing the soil of understanding and bridging the chasms of difference. Let the shoots of integrity pierce the shadows of deceit, illuminating the path towards truth and fostering trust in the darkest corners.

And let the blooms of accountability burst forth, vibrant reminders that our choices, though personal, resonate in the wider world, each action a ripple in the pond of existence. In their journeys towards responsible living, our daughters become not just architects of their own destinies, but stewards of a collective future, wielding the tools of empathy, integrity, and accountability to cultivate a world where every individual flourishes, empowered by the knowledge that their choices, like seeds scattered with love and intention, have the power to blossom into a world where responsibility isn't just a burden, but a shared song, sung in harmonies of action and echoed in the whispers of a collective conscience.

For in their dedication to living well, we find our own purpose, in their empathy our solace, and in their unwavering commitment to a righteous path, we glimpse the dawning of a future where responsibility isn't an afterthought, but a birthright, woven into the very fabric of our being. A future where daughters and mothers, hand in hand, tend the garden of character, ensuring not just their own individual growth, but the flourishing of a world where empathy paints the horizon with vibrant hues of understanding, integrity lights the way with beacons of truth, and accountability becomes the chorus that guides us, together, towards a dawn where every choice, every action, every life ripples outwards, transforming the world into a symphony of responsible living, one note at a time.

Chapter 11: Finding Their Voice: Amplifying The Chorus Of Courage And Conviction

Imagine a world where girls' voices resonate with fearless conviction, echoing in the halls of power, in the whispers of quiet classrooms, and in the vibrant tapestry of diverse opinions. A world where their beliefs, not silenced by shyness or societal expectations, ignite positive change, challenge injustices, and weave a stronger fabric of society. This is the world we strive to create for our daughters – a world where they find their voice, use it boldly, and stand tall as advocates for themselves and the causes they hold dear.

Cultivating Courage, Dispelling Fear:

Our daughters navigate a world that often underestimates the power of a young girl's voice. Help them dismantle the walls of fear, the insecurities whispering doubt in their ears. Encourage open dialogue, creating a safe space where their opinions are valued, celebrated, and respectfully debated. Listen actively, without judgment, fostering an environment where their voices can bloom without the fear of withering under criticism. Remember, silenced voices cannot lead change; encourage your daughter to raise her voice with confidence, knowing that her words hold weight and deserve to be heard.

Beyond Words, The Language of Action:

Empower your daughter to transform her beliefs into action. Encourage her to engage in causes she cares about, whether it's volunteering at an animal shelter, advocating for environmental protection, or raising awareness about social justice issues. Guide her in researching, planning, and implementing projects that give voice to her passion and make a tangible difference in the world. Remember, action amplifies words; help your daughter turn her convictions into catalysts for positive change.

Role Models of Resilience, Champions of Change:

Expose your daughter to stories of inspiring women who defied expectations and used their voices to challenge the status quo. Share narratives of activists, artists, scientists, and everyday heroes who dared to speak their truth and create ripples of change. Let these stories be living testaments to the power of a voice used with purpose, reminding your daughter that she too can rise above societal constraints and leave her mark on the world.

Beyond Walls, Building Bridges of Communication:

Teach your daughter the art of respectful communication, of expressing her opinions with clarity and conviction while acknowledging and appreciating differing perspectives. Encourage her to engage in constructive dialogue, listen actively to opposing viewpoints, and build bridges of understanding rather than walls of division. Remember, effective communication paves the way for progress; equip your daughter with the tools to navigate conversations productively and contribute to a world where diverse voices come together to create positive change.

Navigating the Storm, Facing Resistance with Grace:

The road to finding your voice is not always paved with sunshine. Your daughter may face resistance, criticism, and attempts to silence her. Prepare her for these challenges, reminding her that courage often lies in speaking up when it's difficult, not when it's easy. Teach her to navigate criticism with grace and resilience, using it as an opportunity to refine her arguments and strengthen her conviction. Remember, doubt and opposition can be fertile ground for growth; guide your daughter to weather the storms, emerge stronger, and let her voice rise above the din of disagreement.

Beyond Self, Championing the Chorus of Others:

Encourage your daughter to become an advocate not just for herself, but for others whose voices may be unheard or silenced. Teach her the power of solidarity, of raising her voice in support of marginalized communities, and challenging systemic injustices. Show her how to use her platform, however small, to amplify the voices of those who struggle to be heard and champion causes that promote equality and justice for all. Remember, true power lies in using your voice for the collective good; inspire your daughter to be a chorus leader, lifting the voices of others and creating a symphony of collective change.

Together, Amplifying the Symphony of Change:

In their journeys towards finding their voices, we find our own, in their conviction our inspiration, and in their unwavering commitment to speaking up, we witness the promise of a world where girls don't just whisper their dreams, but shout them from the rooftops. Together, let us raise daughters who break free from the shackles of silence, who speak their truth with confidence, and use their voices not just to navigate their own paths, but to illuminate the way for others.

So let the voices rise, not muffled by fear, but amplified by courage. Let the debates fill the air, not with animosity, but with the vibrant hum of diverse perspectives. Let the challenges met with resistance be transformed into opportunities for growth, turning opposition into fuel for stronger convictions.

And let the chorus of change ring out, not from a single soloist, but from a magnificent symphony of empowered girls, united in their purpose, unwavering in their beliefs, and determined to weave their voices into the tapestry of a world where every opinion resonates with meaning, every injustice finds its challenger, and every individual, young or old, finds the courage to speak their truth and contribute to the vibrant melody of a more just, equitable, and compassionate world. In their voices, we find our own echoes, in their courage our strength, and in their unwavering commitment to speak truth to power, we glimpse the dawning of a future where silence is not an option, where girls stand shoulder-to-shoulder, voices intertwined, chanting the chorus of change, not just for themselves, but for the collective good.

For in their stories of voices found and used with purpose, we find our own liberation, in their defiance our inspiration, and in their symphony of empowered voices, we hear the triumphant anthem of a future where daughters and mothers, hand in hand, raise their voices, not as weapons, but as torches illuminating the path towards a world where every opinion matters, every dream finds its voice, and every girl discovers the transformative power of a voice used with conviction, a voice that can move mountains, shatter glass ceilings, and rewrite the narrative of a world ready to listen, ready to change, and ready to embrace the full, unmuted chorus of empowered young women, ready to sing their song and leave their indelible mark on the world.

Chapter 12: Nurturing A Growth Mindset: Cultivating The Garden Of Resilience And Learning

Imagine a garden where challenges are not weeds, but fertilizer, where mistakes are not wilted blooms, but opportunities for growth, and where setbacks are not storms that uproot, but gentle rains that nourish. This is the garden of a growth mindset, a fertile landscape where our daughters learn to embrace failures as stepping stones, setbacks as detours, and challenges as invitations to blossom anew. As mothers, our role is to become gardeners, tilling the soil of their spirits, planting the seeds of resilience, and nurturing the unwavering belief that even the sturdiest oak grows from a tiny, vulnerable seed.

Planting the Seeds of Belief:

The bedrock of a growth mindset is the fundamental belief that intelligence and abilities are not fixed, but flexible. Teach your daughter that effort leads to growth, that challenges present opportunities to learn, and that mistakes are inevitable stepping stones on the path to mastery. Celebrate her dedication, not just her successes, and emphasize the importance of the journey, not just the destination. Remind her that even the most accomplished individuals stumble, fall, and learn along the way, making the journey all the more enriching.

Watering the Roots of Perseverance:

Obstacles are inevitable on the path to any goal. Encourage your daughter to develop the grit and determination to face them head-on. Celebrate her perseverance, her willingness to try again, her ability to adapt and find new solutions. Help her reframe challenges as opportunities to learn and grow, teaching her that resilience is not the absence of setbacks, but the ability to bounce back stronger from each hurdle.

Nourishing the Blooms of Learning:

Embrace mistakes as fertilizer, not weeds. Teach your daughter to view them as valuable learning experiences, opportunities to discover her strengths and weaknesses, and refine her approach.

Encourage her to analyze her mistakes, learn from them, and use them as stepping stones to future success. Foster a curiosity about failure, a willingness to dissect it, understand it, and use it as a tool for growth. Remember, mistakes don't define us; they refine us.

Pruning the Weeds of Negativity:

Negative self-talk can choke the seeds of a growth mindset. Help your daughter identify and challenge negative thought patterns. Encourage her to replace "I can't" with "I'm learning" and "I'm not good at this" with "I'm still figuring it out." Celebrate her progress, no matter how small, and remind her that consistent effort, not innate talent, is the secret ingredient to success.

Beyond the Garden Walls, Cultivating a Growth Mindset in Action:

Help your daughter apply the principles of a growth mindset beyond the classroom or the playing field. Encourage her to tackle new challenges, learn new skills, and step outside her comfort zone. Celebrate her willingness to experiment, her openness to feedback, and her eagerness to grow in all aspects of her life. Remember, a growth mindset is not just about academics; it's about embracing life as a continuous learning journey.

Weathering the Storms: Reframing Setbacks and Fostering Self-Compassion:

Even the most fertile gardens experience storms. When your daughter faces a setback, be a beacon of light and support. Help her reframe the situation, focusing on what she can learn and how she can move forward. Guide her towards self-compassion, reminding her that everyone experiences setbacks, and it's okay to feel disappointment without drowning in it.

Beyond Self, Sharing the Seeds of Growth:

A growth mindset is not just for our daughters; it's a gift we can share with the world. Encourage your daughter to become a mentor, supporting others in their learning journeys and celebrating their efforts. Let her role model the principles of a growth mindset, demonstrating the power of perseverance, resilience, and a constant quest for learning. Remember, by sharing the seeds of growth, we cultivate a thriving forest of resilience and optimism, where everyone flourishes under the sun of their own potential.

Together, Cultivating a Forest of Potential:

In their journeys towards embracing a growth mindset, we find our own, in their resilience our strength, and in their unwavering belief in the power of learning, we witness the promise of a brighter future. Together, let us raise daughters who not only weather the storms of life but thrive in them, who see challenges as opportunities to bloom, and who approach every setback with the unwavering conviction that "I can't" is just a stepping stone on the path to "I will."

So let the gardens flourish, not just within them, but outwards, into the community, weaving tendrils of resilience and a thirst for learning that bind us together in a shared love of growth. Let the roots of perseverance burrow deep, anchoring them in the face of adversity and providing the nourishment for their dreams to blossom. Let the blooms of self-compassion burst forth, vibrant reminders that mistakes are not blemishes, but brushstrokes in the vibrant masterpiece of their lives. And let the tendrils of inspiration reach out, sharing the seeds of a growth mindset with others, transforming the landscape of our world from barren fields of doubt to a thriving forest of endless possibility, where every individual learns, adapts, and blooms anew, fueled by the knowledge that challenges are fertilizer, setbacks are detours, and the journey of learning is a magnificent symphony played on the strings of resilience, the drums of curiosity, and the windswept chords of unwavering belief.

For in their stories of embracing a growth mindset, we find our own pathways to evolve, in their perseverance our resilience, and in their unwavering pursuit of learning, we glimpse the dawning of a future where growth isn't a luxury, but a birthright, woven into the very fabric of our being. A future where daughters and mothers, hand in hand, tend the garden of potential, not just for themselves, but for the collective good, ensuring not just their own individual flourishing, but the blossoming of a world where challenges inspire, setbacks redirect, and every moment, from triumph to stumble, becomes a fertile ground for endless learning, endless growth, and a symphony of potential, forever in bloom.

Conclusion: Embracing The Whirlwind, Cultivating Strength: Raising Strong, Empowered Girls In The 21St Century

Motherhood in the 21st century is a dance on a tightrope woven from digital threads and social complexities. Raising strong, empowered girls in this whirlwind landscape can feel like navigating a maze blindfolded, each turn revealing new challenges, each decision tinged with the weight of shaping who they'll become.

But fear not, mothers-of-daughters, for this journey, though daunting, is also breathtakingly beautiful. We stand at the precipice of a future where girls are not confined to pre-ordained boxes, but equipped to rewrite their own narratives, shatter glass ceilings, and redefine what it means to be strong, compassionate, and empowered.

This book has been a compass, a lantern held aloft in the shadows, offering tools and resources to guide you through the labyrinth.

We've explored the importance of open communication, the resilience built from navigating challenges, the strength found in setting boundaries, and the courage needed to raise your voice. We've planted the seeds of empathy, nurtured the sapling of integrity, and cultivated the garden of a growth mindset.

Yet, tools and resources are just the mortar; the bricks are built from your unwavering love, your fierce support, and your unwavering belief in their potential. Trust their intuition, celebrate their unique quirks, and guide them with gentle hands and open hearts. Be their fiercest advocate, their safe haven, and their loudest cheerleader. Remember, you are not alone in this journey; a whole chorus of mothers, daughters, and supporters stands beside you, their voices echoing your own, their experiences lending strength to your convictions.

There will be stumbles, tears, and moments of doubt, nights spent whispering reassurances and mornings wiping away anxieties. But amidst it all, there will be triumphs, bursts of laughter, and moments of breathtaking resilience that leave you awestruck by the sheer force of their spirit. These are the moments that weave the tapestry of our motherhood, the threads of challenge and joy intertwined, creating a masterpiece of love and light.

This critical time of raising strong, empowered girls is not just about shaping individuals; it's about shaping the future. By equipping our daughters with the tools to navigate this complex world, we are building a generation of women who are leaders, changemakers, and architects of a more just and equitable society. We are planting the seeds of a future where diversity is celebrated, empathy reigns, and compassion binds us together.

So, let us walk into this future with heads held high, hearts overflowing with hope, and eyes sparkling with the confidence that our daughters will not just survive, but thrive. Let us embrace the whirlwind, not with fear, but with the conviction that in the chaos lies the potential for incredible beauty, for in raising strong, empowered girls, we are not just shaping mothers and daughters, but co-creating a world where every woman, young and old, can stand tall and sing her own powerful song.

Remember, mothers-of-daughters, you are not alone. We are a tapestry woven from countless threads of love, a symphony of voices raised in support, a chorus of hope echoing through the generations. Together, let us continue this dance, step by step, hand in hand, raising strong, empowered girls who will change the world, one powerful leap at a time.

The future is theirs to write, and ours to illuminate with the unwavering belief that their strength, their compassion, and their unwavering spirits will light the way to a brighter tomorrow. So let the story unfold, the future unfurl, and let us embrace the joy, the challenges, and the breathtaking privilege of raising strong, empowered girls in the 21st century. For in their journey, we find our own, in their voices our strength, and in their hopeful eyes, we glimpse the dawn of a world where every girl, every woman, every mother, and daughter can rise, flourish, and write their own unforgettable tale of strength, grace, and the unwavering power of being a girl, a woman, a force to be reckoned with, in this magnificent, ever-evolving landscape called the 21st century.

www.ingramcontent.com/pod-product-compliance
Lightning Source LLC
Chambersburg PA
CBHW070814250726
48662CB00004B/2042